A Chef's Guide to Cooking with Essential Oils

Scentfanatic  Publishing™

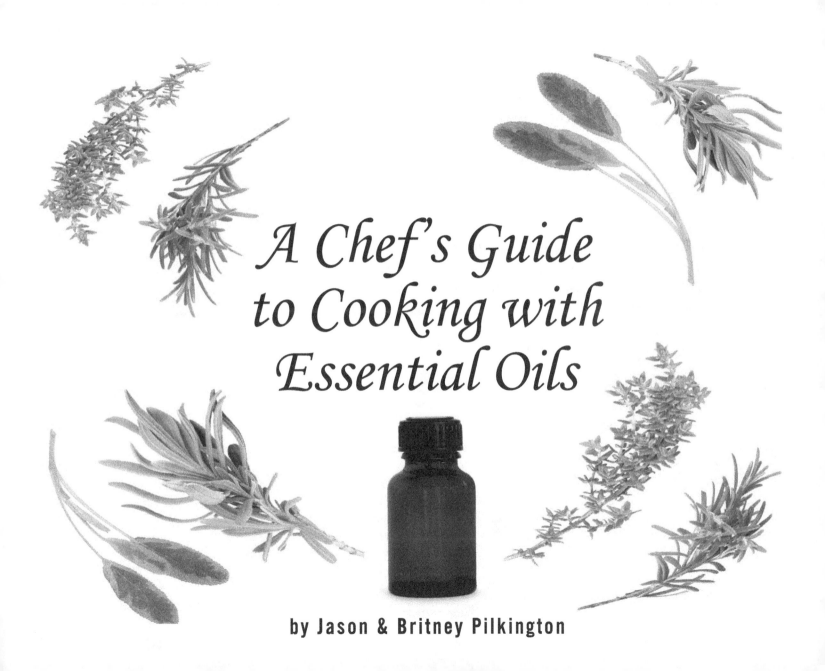

A Chef's Guide to Cooking with Essential Oils

by Jason & Britney Pilkington

A Chef's Guide to Cooking with Essential Oils
By Jason & Britney Pilkington
Copyright © 2015 by Jason & Britney Pilkington
All rights reserved.

Layout, Design and cover: Clyde L. Pilkington III
Image credits:
canstockphoto/marilyna
canstockphoto/arrakeshh
canstockphoto/olenayemchuk

ISBN-13: 978-1-62904-041-7
Published by: ScentfanaticPublishing™

For information on Scentfanatic Publishing™ releases, visit:
www.ScentfanaticPublishing.com

Printed in the United States of America.

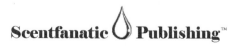

We are proud to aid you in your journey in incorporating essential oils into every day of your life! We have been incredibly blessed by Young Living's essential oils. They are the only company on the market offering oils that we feel comfortable recommending to you for use in the kitchen. They have the exceptional quality necessary for internal use. If you have not yet joined Young Living, you are welcome to use our ID: 611218

To gain a better understanding of the therapeutic essential oils, we recommend purchasing a desk reference. Our personal favorites are the "Essential Oils Desk Reference" by Life Science Publishing and the "Reference Guide for Essential Oils" by Connie and Alan Higley.

> *"Thy God, hath anointed thee with the oil of gladness above thy fellows. All thy garments smell of myrrh, and aloes, and cassia, out of the ivory palaces, whereby they have made thee glad."* (Psalms 45:7,8)

Table of Contents

Introduction

We first began using essential oils for a healthier, happier life back in 2002, when we were introduced to Young Living. In 2007, Jason attended Le Cordon Bleu College of Culinary Arts in Las Vegas, and not long afterward we came to realize that we could use the oils in the kitchen! With his new found culinary knowledge, it was easy to substitute oils for other ingredients in recipes and find new applications for them. Through our experimentation we found that we were experiencing new flavors! For example, lemon essential oil lends a different flavor than lemon extract or lemon zest can. At the time, we had not heard of anyone else cooking with oils, so we were excited about our discovery. (Young Living was not yet posting recipes in the monthly newsletter, and we had never even looked at Youngliving.com). In 2012 we started the facebook page A Chef's Guide to Young Living Essential Oils, just for fun! We have posted recipes there sporadically as a hobby. Since 2010, Jason has been a stay-at-home dad and personal chef to our family. We now have two children and our own business, but we try our best to experiment with new recipes at least a few times per month. Many people have approached us at the Young Living convention and left us facebook messages asking us to write a cookbook. We have also heard a lot of requests for an herb/essential oil conversion chart. We have worked hard to provide you here with both. Please enjoy!

Why Use Essential Oils in the Kitchen?

So why would you substitute an essential oil for an herb? Dried herbs are cheaper, right? If you consider the fact that one drop of oregano essential oil can be substituted for three tablespoons of dried herbs, and a 15 ML bottle of oregano contains around two hundred and fifty drops, that may not be the case with most herbs. The average shelf life for dried herbs is six months for ideal potency and flavor. The shelf life of a bottle of pure, steam-distilled essential oil is thousands of years! Citrus oils have a shelf life of about one year.

Pure essential oils have been used since ancient times to promote good health and aid in healing a variety of ailments. Distillation equipment has been found dating back to 3500 B.C.E. Thirty-three different kinds of essential oils are mentioned over six hundred times in the Bible. Today, many people are realizing the benefits of using pure essential oils. Research in the past one hundred years has corroborated what our ancestors knew about the benefits they provide. Essential oils can be used topically on the skin, diffused into the air, inhaled from the bottle, or taken internally. So why not expand the applications by using them in your food? Essential oils are used in food in very small amounts due to their potency, but they will provide you with beneficial molecules. Remember, one drop of essential oil may contain up to 40, 000,000,000,000,000,000 (40 quintillion) molecules! It is important to be aware that heating your food too hot will destroy those molecules. We avoid damage by checking the temperature of our food.

For example: when we add oils to soups, we wait until the very end, after the heat has been turned off. Pure, steam-distilled essential oils are safe up to approximately 260 degrees Fahrenheit because most oils reach this temperature at some point during distillation. Citrus oils, which are expressed and contain larger molecules than steam-distilled oils, should not be heated above 100 degrees Fahrenheit to preserve their health benefits. But the heat does not destroy the flavor, so you may still use essential oils in things that get above these temperatures. Many people have asked us if essential oils will lose their therapeutic value if they put them in hot tea. This is not a problem you have to worry about unless you drink your tea boiling hot. In fact, an essential oil in tea is a wonderful application. You might ask, what if I am putting the oil in something that is going to be frozen? Well, freezing will not hurt your essential oil at all. So feel free to add it to granita, ice cream, popsicles, etc. Another thing we would like to mention is that the chemistry of some essential oils can change when added to water. Oils with high ester content (lavender being the only one used in water in this book) may have their chemistry slightly altered when they come in contact with water, altering the therapeutic value of the oil.

Essential Oil Safety in the Kitchen

We believe the most important safety advice we can give you is to use the purest essential oils available. Not only do we want to avoid the petrochemicals and synthetic ingredients included in many essential oils on the market, but we want every healing molecule available to us that is found in a true "therapeutic- grade" essential oil. As of right now, the only essential oil brand we trust is Young Living. Some other brands claim to be better, but we have tried them out, and so have our friends. In our opinion, no other company has yet achieved Young Living's high level of quality.

Always remember that pure essential oils are very potent. Did you know that one drop of peppermint essential oil is equal in strength to about twenty peppermint tea bags? In cooking we generally use only 1-20 drops in any one recipe, with citrus oils needing the highest number of drops. As long as you are using truly pure oils, you do not need to be concerned about the safety of these small amounts in your food. We have had many people ask us, "If you consume a photo-sensitive oil, like lemon, can you get skin discoloration if you get UV exposure after eating it?" The answer is no! This is not something to worry about. Some "hot" oils like cinnamon or clove can irritate sensitive skins. As long as you are adding drops straight from the bottle into your food, you should not have to worry about contact with your skin. But if it happens, and irritation occurs, simply grab some olive oil and rub a drop or two on the affected area.

You should consult with your doctor before ingesting certain oils if you are pregnant or nursing. Of the oils used in the recipes in this book, some of the ones to avoid include nutmeg, tarragon, basil, sage, rosemary, and fennel.

Substitution & Conversion

Regarding substitution, there are a few things to keep in mind when you want to replace a dried herb, extract, etc. with an essential oil in a recipe.

An essential oil's flavor may differ slightly from the herb of the same name. It may not always be the best choice to substitute an oil for an herb. For example, if you substitute lemon essential oil for lemon juice, you will not get any of the juice's tart flavor in your recipe. If you would still like to add oil as well, you can adjust the recipe. Of course, as we mentioned in our introduction, we find that essential oils offer new and exciting flavors! Just experiment and have fun.

Just as you may adjust herbs, salt, and pepper "to taste," we recommend doing the same with your oils. Some preparations, such as a batter containing raw eggs, for example, you may not want to taste. For such cases (and of course as a general guideline for any situation), we have put together a conversion chart that you can find on page 17.

You might want to keep that herb for the sake of color and texture! Sometimes the brown flecks of cinnamon or the green flakes of oregano will be missed. Food is an art form, and some herbs have visual effects that should not be left out. If you would like to substitute essential oil for some of a dried herb, just decrease the amount you use of the herb and start with a small amount of oil, then adjust the drops to taste.

As you will see in the conversion chart that follows, the essential oil is listed on the left side of the chart and at the top are the measurements of the herb that the essential oil is being substituted for. When we started to create a list with different amounts of essential oil for lemon juice, lemon extract, and lemon zest for example, the list became incredibly lengthy and we wished to simplify. We designed this chart to be a guideline, not exact measurements. We taste tested the different herb forms and how they correspond with the essential oil, and chose what we felt is the closest. Most often times the dried herb form is stronger in flavor than the fresh. This chart recommends the same amount of essential oil for both preparations. Start with these amounts then you can always add more essential oil to taste. We have found that not everyone likes the same flavor strengths. Just as you would do in any recipe, start with a very small amount and adjust accordingly; you can add more much easier than you can take some out!

You will notice the abbreviation "TPD" on this chart. This stands for "Toothpick Dip". Sometimes 1 drop of essential oil is a little too much! We recommend that when you first start using oils in the kitchen, you start with using toothpick dips only, so you can get an idea of how strong you like your flavors. There are two ways to do this. We like to put the toothpick down the air vent in the orifice reducer of the bottle (be sure there is enough oil in the bottle so that it is getting on the toothpick), pull it out, then use the toothpick to stir whatever you are adding the oil to. Alternatively, you may remove the orifice reducer first.

Conversion Chart

	1/4 Teaspoon	1/2 Teaspoon	1 Teaspoon	1 Tablespoon
Basil	2 TPD	1 drop	2 drops	4 drops
Black Pepper	1 drop	2 drops	4 drops	8 drops
Bay Laurel	1 leaf = 1 drop	2 leaf = 2 drops	3 leaf = 3 drops	4 leaf = 4 drops
Cinnamon Bark	1 TPD	1 stick = 2 TPD	2 sticks = 1 drop	3 sticks = 2 drops
Clove	1 clove = 1 TPD	2 cloves = 2 TPD	3 cloves = 4 TPD	4 cloves = 1 drop
Celery Seed	1 TPD	2 TPD	1 drop	2 drops
Cardamom	1 TPD	2 TPD	1 drop	2 drops
Coriander	1 TPD	2 TPD	3 TPD	1 drop
Dill	1 TPD	2 TPD	1 drop	3 drops
Grapefruit	1 drop	2 drops	4 drops	8 drops
Lime	1 drop	2 drops	4 drops	8 drops
Lemon	1 drop	2 drops	4 drops	8 drops
Lemongrass	1 stalk = 1 drop	2 stalks = 2 drops	3 stalks = 3 drops	4 stalks = 4 drops
Nutmeg	2 TPD	1 drop	2 drops	4 drops
Orange	1 drop	2 drops	4 drops	8 drops
Oregano	1 TPD	2 TPD	1 drop	2 drops
Peppermint	2 TPD	3 TPD	1 drop	3 drops
Rose	1 TPD	2 TPD	3 TPD	1 drop
Rosemary	2 TPD	1 drop	2 drops	4 drops
Sage	2 TPD	1 drop	2 drops	4 drops
Tarragon	1 TPD	2 TPD	3 TPD	2 drops
Thyme	1 TPD	2 TPD	1 drop	2 drops

Breakfast

Overnight Oats & Quinoa

Of course you can make this in a large saucepan on the stove, if you don't want to use a crock-pot. Cook over low heat until done, about 20 minutes.

1 1/2 cup old fashioned rolled oats

1/2 cup quinoa, rinsed

1/2 cup raisins and/or dried cranberries, dried cherries, dried goji berries, etc.

4 cups water

1 teaspoon salt

1/8 cup agave syrup

1 drop cinnamon essential oil

1 drop nutmeg essential oil

2 toothpick dips cardamom

Combine all ingredients except for the agave and essential oils, in a crockpot. Cook 6-8 hours on low. Before serving, mix essential oils with the agave in a small bowl. Pour agave/oil mixture over oats and combine. Adjust sweetness with brown sugar, maple syrup, yacon syrup, stevia, or more agave. Serve with chopped nuts and milk (optional). This recipe serves 6-8 people.

Skillet Peppers & Eggs

½ cup extra virgin olive oil

1 large onion, sliced thin

1 red bell pepper, cut into strips

1 yellow bell pepper, cut into strips

salt & pepper

2 drops bay laurel essential oil

1 drop thyme essential oil

2 tablespoons fresh parsley, chopped

2 tablespoons fresh cilantro, chopped

1 28 ounce can, diced tomatoes

approximately 1 cup water

8 eggs

In a large skillet, cook onions in olive oil over medium high heat for about 5 minutes. Add peppers and cook for 5 more minutes. Add tomatoes, salt and pepper. Reduce heat and cook on low for 15 minutes, adding water from time to time to maintain a sauce consistency. Turn heat to lowest setting. Add the essential oils and stir to combine. Make 4 wells in the sauce and crack two eggs into each hole. Cover with a lid and cook over the lowest heat setting until eggs are cooked, about 15 minutes. Be sure the sauce does not simmer. Remove from heat. Sprinkle parsley and cilantro over before serving. Serves 4 people.

Gingerbread Waffles

This is a delightful variation on the average plain waffle.

1 cup (4 1/4 ounces) all-purpose flour

1 cup whole wheat flour (4 ounces)

2 teaspoons baking powder

1/2 teaspoon baking soda

1/2 teaspoon salt

3 drops ginger essential oil

2 drops nutmeg essential oil

2 drops clove essential oil

4 eggs

6 tablespoons butter (3 ounces)

1 cup milk

1/2 cup (4 ounces) sour cream

3 tablespoons molasses (2 1/4 ounces)

Preheat your iron while you make the waffle batter. Whisk together the flours, baking powder, baking soda, salt and oils. In a separate bowl, whisk together the eggs, melted butter, milk, sour cream, and molasses. Add the wet to the dry mixture ingredients, mixing until just combined (The batter will be lumpy). Cook the waffles as directed in the instructions that came with your waffle iron. Makes 10 waffles.

Put the Lime in the Coconut Granola

This granola recipe is very customizable! Swap the coconut oil for olive oil and agave for maple syrup or honey. Use different nuts, try different oils, and even add chocolate chips, raisins, or dried cherries! Add the chocolate and dried fruit at the end after baking. Here, we use lime essential oil which will lose its therapeutic value at 100°F, but we cannot cook the granola that low. If you are using a steam distilled oil, feel free to bake the granola at 250°F for about 1 hour instead of the time mentioned in the recipe.

1 large beaten egg white

3 cups old-fashioned rolled oats

1 1/2 cups chopped raw almonds

1 1/2 cups unsweetened coconut

1/2 cup agave syrup

1/4 cup warmed coconut oil

1 1/2 teaspoons kosher salt

16 drops lime essential oil

Preheat your oven to 300°F. Combine the lime essential oil and agave in a large bowl. Add the remaining ingredients, then toss to combine. Spread the mixture out on a rimmed baking sheet. Bake granola, stirring every 10 minutes, until golden brown and dry, about 40 minutes. Let cool on the baking sheet. Store the granola airtight at room temperature.

EO Infused Yogurt

There are so many ways you can customize this recipe. We also like adding lemon essential oil and adding fresh strawberries. When trying a different oil, start with a very small amount and add more to taste.

1/2 cup plain Greek yogurt,

1 toothpick dip ocotea essential oil

1 tablespoon honey

In a small bowl, combine the yogurt and essential oil and drizzle the honey over the top. Serve cold, and with granola if desired. Serves 1.

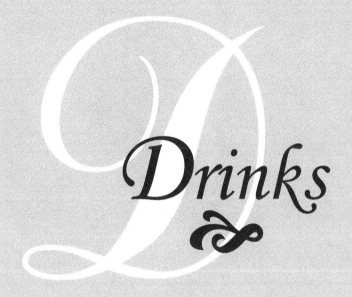

Drinks

Lavender Lemonade

7 lemons, juiced

2 limes, juiced

5-6 drops lavender oil

12 drops lemon oil

14 cups water

1 1/2 cup agave nectar

Mix all ingredients together in a gallon jug or pitcher and chill.

Citus Ginger Refresher

4 medium oranges, halved

1 medium grapefruit, halved

2 medium lemons, halved

1 large lime, halved

1 drop each of lemon, orange, tangerine, grapefruit and ginger essential oils

Use a juicer to juice the fruit into a small pitcher. Add essential oils to juice and stir before serving.

Chocolate Smoothie with Orange Essential Oil

1 cup almond milk (or coconut milk, or rice milk)

1 tablespoon cocoa powder

2 drops orange essential oil

A few ice cubes (amount optional)

1 fresh banana

1/2 teaspoon vanilla

1 tablespoon coconut oil

Agave nectar to sweeten (optional)

Add all ingredients in a blender and puree until smooth.

Immune Booster Drink

1 cup hot water

1-2 teaspoon raw honey

1 teaspoon Bragg's Raw Apple Cider Vinegar

2 drops of lemon or orange essential oil

1 drop Young Living Thieves essential oil

Combine all ingredients in an 8 ounce glass. Stir before drinking.

Banana, Berry, & Orange Oil Smoothie

1 cup berries (raspberries, blueberries, blackberries, and/or strawberries)

1 banana

1/4 cup orange juice

1/4 cup vanilla almond milk

1 cup ice cubes

2-4 drops orange essential oil

Combine all ingredients in a blender and puree until smooth.

EO Gin & Tonic

There could certainly be a whole book on essential oils in cocktails. Here we are including one recipe that we use, that can give you an idea of how to work oils into drinks such as this one.

5 or 6 ice cubes

3 ounces gin

4 ounces tonic water (we like Vling or Fever Tree)

1 toothpick dip juniper essential oil

2 drops lime essential oil

lime wedge (optional, for garnish)

Place ice cubes in a glass, add the gin and lime essential oil. Add the tonic water. Use a toothpick dipped in juniper essential oil to stir. Garnish with a lime wedge if desired.

Appetizers, Snacks & Side Dishes

Cherry Quinoa Nut Bars

Why pay the money for pre-packaged energy bars, when you can make your own? This recipe makes about 12 of them (depending on how big you cut them). Feel free to swap out any of the nuts and seeds with whatever other nuts and seeds you have on hand.

1 cup chopped raw almonds

1/2 cup quinoa, rinsed

1/4 cup raw sunflower seeds

1/4 cup whole flax seed

1 cup dried cherries

2 tablespoons brown rice syrup

1 tablespoon water

1/2 teaspoon sea salt

1 drop cassia or cinnamon essential oil

Lightly coat an 8 x 8 inch baking pan with cooking spray. Line the pan with parchment paper, leaving overhang on all sides. You may leave the nuts and seeds raw, or you can combine the almonds, quinoa, and sunflower seeds on a cookie sheet, and toast lightly in a 350 °F oven, about 5 minutes. After you remove them, lower the oven temperature to 200 degrees F.

Combine the cherries, brown rice syrup, salt, essential oil and 1 tablespoon of water in a food processor and process until smooth, scraping down the sides if needed. Transfer nuts and cherry mixture to a medium bowl and combine thoroughly. Press the mixture down firmly into the prepared pan. If the mixture is not packed tightly enough, your bars will not stay together. (We use a flat-bottomed drinking glass to help with this.)

Bake the bars until they are no longer sticky, about 25-30 minutes. Let cool in the pan, then, remove the bars by lifting the parchment up and out of the pan by the overhang. Cut into bars. We recommend wrapping these individually in plastic wrap. They will last for 2-3 weeks at room temperature this way.

Fruity Oat Snacks

These little snacks are gluten-free, egg free, dairy free, and sugar free. They are very simple to make and they taste great!

3 ripe bananas, mashed

1/3 cup applesauce (we made our own and left it nice and chunky)

2 cups oats (gluten free)

¼ cup almond milk

½ cup raisins, craisins, or dried cherries

1 teaspoon vanilla

1 drop cinnamon essential oil

Mix all ingredients in a large bowl. Scoop the dough by the tablespoon full onto a greased baking sheet, or one lined with parchment paper. Bake at 350 °F for 15-20 minutes, until they feel firm to the touch.

Bulgur Stuffed Swiss Chard

In a large pot of boiling salted water, blanch the chard leaves until bright green, about 1 minute. Drain the leaves and rinse under cold water. Drain again, then carefully pat the leaves dry with paper towels.

In a medium saucepan, bring the 2 cups water to a rolling boil. Add the bulgur, give it a stir, then turn off the heat. Cover immediately and let stand until the water has been absorbed and the bulgur is tender, about 15 minutes.

In a skillet, heat the 3 tablespoons of oil. Add the onion and cook over moderate heat until translucent, about 4 minutes. Add the diced tomato and cook until sizzling, about 1 minute. Remove from the heat. Combine the olive oil and essential oils in a small bowl, set aside. Stir the bulgur, red pepper flakes, and parsley into the tomato and onion mixture. Drizzle the essential oil mixture over and stir to combine. Season to taste with salt and pepper.

Spread a chard leaf out on a work surface, overlapping the leaf to fill the space where the rib was. Mound 2-3 tablespoons of the filling on the lower third of the leaf. Bring the lower end of the leaf up and over the filling and roll up tightly, folding in the sides as you go. Repeat with the remaining leaves and filling. Arrange the stuffed leaves on a platter. Drizzle with oil, season with salt, and serve.

24 medium Swiss chard leaves, stems and ribs removed, (about 2 bunches)

1 cup coarse bulgur (about 6 ounces)

2 cups boiling water

3 tablespoons canola or vegetable oil

1 medium onion, chopped fine

2 teaspoons crushed red pepper flakes (optional, but recommended)

2 plum tomatoes, diced into 1/4-inch pieces

2 tablespoons fresh parsley, chopped fine

1 tablespoon extra-virgin olive oil, plus more for drizzling

22 drops lemon essential oil

2 drops dill essential oil

1 drop peppermint essential oil

salt

freshly ground pepper

Spinach and Artichoke Dip

1 12-16oz bag chopped frozen spinach, thawed

1 cup chopped canned or frozen artichoke hearts, thawed

1 8 ounce package Neufchatel or cream cheese

1/4 cup grated parmesan cheese

1/2 cup grated Monterey Jack cheese

1/2 cup shredded white sharp cheddar cheese

1/4 cup heavy cream

1/4 cup chicken stock

1 teaspoon cumin

1/4 teaspoon salt

2 garlic cloves, minced

2 drops black pepper essential oil

1 drop coriander oil

Combine all ingredients except for the essential oils in a large saucepan or Dutch oven. Cook over low heat, stirring occasionally until dip is smooth and heated through. Remove from heat, and add essential oils. Stir to combine. This can also be made in a slow-cooker.

Creamy Cucumber Dill Dip

1 seedless cucumber, chopped into chunks

4 tablespoons sour cream or plain Greek yogurt (or a mix of the two)

1 tablespoon olive oil

1 tablespoon distilled white vinegar

1 drop dill essential oil

1/4 teaspoon garlic powder

2 drops black pepper oil

salt to taste

Combine all ingredients in a blender, and puree until smooth. Chill in the refrigerator, or serve immediately. Serve with crackers, flatbread, and vegetable crudités.

Avocado & Pea Crostini

2 tablespoons extra virgin olive oil

juice from ½ a lime

1 teaspoon finely chopped mint

4 drops lime essential oil

1 drop tarragon essential oil

1 dash cayenne pepper

1 dash salt and freshly ground pepper

1 small avocado, diced ½ inch or smaller

4 small slices of bread, crackers, or flatbread

2 tablespoons frozen peas, thawed

In a small bowl, whisk together the olive oil, lime juice, mint, essential oils, cayenne pepper, salt, and pepper. Stir in the avocado and peas with a fork, smashing the avocado slightly. Spoon on top of the bread, crackers, or flatbread. Serves 2-4 people.

Spinach and Feta Puffs

1 10-ounce package frozen chopped spinach, thawed

1/2 cup crumbled feta

1/4 cup minced onion

1 tablespoon olive oil

1 drop dill essential oil

2 drops black pepper essential oil

1 teaspoon minced garlic

salt

2 large eggs

1 sheet frozen puff pastry
    (from a 17.3-ounce package),
    thawed, rolled out to a
    12-inch square, kept chilled

Using your hands, squeeze spinach until dry, forcing out as much water as possible (too much water will make for a soggy filling; you should have about 2/3 cup well-drained spinach). Mix spinach and next 6 ingredients in a medium bowl. Season to taste with salt. In a small bowl, beat 1 egg to blend; fold into spinach mixture.

Cut puff pastry into 3 equal strips. Reserve 1 strip for another use. Cut each remaining strip into 3 squares for a total of 6. Place a square in each muffin cup, pressing into bottom and up sides and leaving corners pointing up. Divide filling among cups. Fold pastry over filling, pressing corners together to meet in center.

Preheat oven to 400°F. Beat remaining egg to blend in a small bowl. Brush pastry with egg wash (this will give the pastry a nice sheen). Bake until pastry is golden brown and puffed, about 25 minutes. Transfer to a wire rack; let puffs cool in pan for 10 minutes. Run a sharp paring knife around pan edges to loosen; turn out puffs onto rack to cool slightly before serving.

Quick Homemade Salsa

This recipe instructs you to let the salsa refrigerate overnight, but of course if you're short on time, a few hours will suffice.

3 cups chopped tomatoes

1/2 cup chopped green bell pepper

1 cup onion, diced

1/4 cup minced fresh cilantro

2 tablespoons fresh lime juice

1 clove garlic, minced

4 teaspoons chopped fresh jalapeno pepper (including seeds)

1/2 teaspoon ground cumin

1/2 teaspoon salt

4 drops black pepper essential oil

1 drop basil essential oil

Stir all ingredients together. Refrigerate overnight to allow flavors to meld. Serve chilled.

Basil and Toasted Pine Nut Hummus

1 cup cooked chickpeas, drained

2 garlic cloves, chopped

2 tablespoons tahini

2 tablespoons lemon juice

1/2 cup extra-virgin olive oil

1 drop basil essential oil

salt

freshly ground black pepper or 1 drop black pepper essential oil

1/2 cup pine nuts

In a food processor, puree the chickpeas, garlic, tahini and lemon juice. Gradually add the olive oil until incorporated. Season the hummus with the basil essential oil, salt and black pepper and scrape it into a bowl. Toast pine nuts in a skillet over low heat until fragrant. Sprinkle pine nuts over the hummus and serve or refrigerate until ready to use.

Jalapeño Lime Popcorn

Depending on the jalapeño you use, this can be very spicy. If you don't want that, remove the seeds from the pepper before adding it to the oil.

8 cups popped popcorn
1/3 cup canola oil
1 small jalapeño, sliced
4 drops lime essential oil
salt

Place the oil in a small saucepan over low heat, add the pepper slices and cook, keeping it below a simmer for 10 minutes. Remove from heat and remove the solids by running the oil through a fine mesh strainer, into a small bowl. Add the lime essential oil to the strained oil. Place the popcorn in a large bowl, slowly drizzle the oil into the popcorn while simultaneously stirring the popcorn with a spatula or wooden spoon to combine. Sprinkle salt over popcorn, combine and then taste, adding more salt to desired strength. Store in an airtight container for up to 1 week.

Orange Coconut Milk Creamsicles

I used full-fat coconut milk for this recipe, but I think you could easily substitute heavy cream or vanilla ice cream for the coconut milk.

12 ounce can full-fat coconut milk

3/4 cup orange juice

1 teaspoon vanilla extract

3 tablespoons honey

4 drops orange oil

1 drop tangerine oil

Combine all the ingredients in a bowl and blend well. Pour the orange mixture into pop molds and freeze for at least 4 hours. To release pops from the mold, run the mold under hot water for a few seconds.

Makes 6 pops

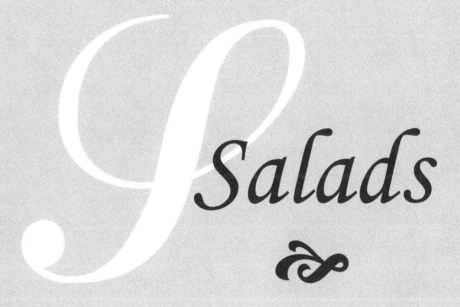

Salads

Warm Cauliflower and Herbed Barley Salad

This is an incredibly satisfying main dish with lots of flavor!

Place barley in a large saucepan; add water to cover by 2". Season with salt. Bring to a boil and cook until tender, 25-30 minutes. Drain, then rinse under cold water. Set aside.

1/2 cup pearled barley

salt

1 tablespoon finely grated lemon zest

15 drops lemon essential oil

2 drops tarragon essential oil

1 tablespoon mayonnaise

1 teaspoon Dijon mustard

6 tablespoons olive oil, divided

freshly ground black pepper

1 head cauliflower, cut into florets

1 15-ounce can Lima or butter beans, rinsed

1/2 cup flat-leaf parsley leaves

Meanwhile, whisk lemon juice, mayonnaise, Dijon mustard, lemon oil, tarragon oil and 5 tablespoons olive oil in a medium bowl until emulsified. Season with salt and pepper; set aside.

Heat remaining 1 tablespoon oil in a large skillet over medium heat. Add cauliflower; cook, turning occasionally, until browned in spots, 10-12 minutes. Add 2 tablespoons water, cover, and cook until just tender, about 2 minutes longer. Season with salt and pepper.

Transfer cauliflower to a large bowl. Add beans, 1/4 cup parsley, and reserved barley. Add dressing. Toss to coat then season to taste with salt and pepper. Garnish with lemon zest (optional), 1/4 cup parsley. Serves 4 -6

Avocado & Tarragon Dressing

1 avocado

2 tablespoons fresh lime juice

1 garlic clove, minced

1/4 cup water

6 tablespoons extra virgin olive oil

1 teaspoon salt

2 drops tarragon essential oil

Combine all ingredients in a blender and blend until smooth. Makes about 1 cup. Serve over mild greens. Vegetables that go well with this dressing include: carrots, artichokes, fresh tomato, cooked beet, and asparagus. Feta cheese is a great addition to this as well.

Barley and Arugula Salad with Beets and Feta

1/4 cup plus 2 tablespoons extra-virgin olive oil; more for drizzling

2 tablespoon white wine vinegar

2 tablespoons coconut or palm sugar

8 drops orange essential oil

2 drops black pepper essential oil

1 bunch arugula

1/4 cup minced shallots

3 medium beets (about 1 bunch), trimmed

1 1/4 cups pearl barley

4 ounces feta, crumbled

2 tablespoons (or more) unseasoned rice vinegar

Whisk 1/4 cup oil, white wine vinegar, sugar, orange and pepper oils in a large bowl to blend; season with salt. Add shallots; mix until completely coated. Cover and chill.

Meanwhile, preheat oven to 375°F. Arrange beets in a small baking dish and drizzle with a little oil. Season with salt and turn beets to coat. Cover with foil. Bake beets until tender when pierced with a thin knife, about 45 minutes. Let cool completely. Peel beets. Cut into 1/4-inch pieces (you should have about 2 cups). Cook barley in a large pot of boiling salted water until just tender, about 45 minutes. Drain barley and spread out on a rimmed baking sheet; let cool completely.

Add beets, barley, arugula and feta to dressing. Drizzle salad with remaining 2 tablespoons oil and 2 tablespoons rice vinegar; fold gently to combine. Season to taste with more rice vinegar, if desired.

Citrus Salad with Rose

This salad takes a little extra work in preparation of the citrus. But trust us, it's worth it! We've put this with the salads, but it would make an excellent dessert as well.

3 grapefruits

3 oranges

3 mandarin, clementine, or blood oranges

3 tablespoons agave

1 drop rose essential oil

¼ cup chopped, toasted hazelnuts or almonds

fresh mint leaves for garnish (optional)

Remove the peel from the grapefruits and oranges with a knife, doing your best to remove all of the white pith. Remove the fruit from between the membranes with a sharp knife, making membrane-free wedges. (This kind of cut is called a "supreme".) Add the citrus to a medium bowl. In a small bowl, combine the agave with 1 drop of rose essential oil, being very careful to only get one drop! Drizzle the agave/rose mixture over the fruit, and very gently toss to combine. Sprinkle nuts over the salad, and garnish with fresh mint

Crushed Beets with Lemon & Dill Vinaigrette

2 pounds mixed small or medium beets, scrubbed

6 tablespoons olive oil, divided, plus more for drizzling

1 drop black pepper essential oil

2 tablespoons finely grated lemon zest

2 tablespoons fresh lemon juice

2 drops dill essential oil

½ cup plain Greek yogurt

flaky sea salt

Preheat oven to 400°F. Divide beets between 2 large sheets of foil. Drizzle beets on each sheet with ½ Tbsp. oil; season with kosher salt and pepper and wrap up foil around beets. Roast on a rimmed baking sheet until tender, 40–50 minutes. Let cool slightly, then, using a paper towel, rub skins from beets (they should slip off easily). Crush beets with the bottom of a small bowl (it's alright if they fall apart).

Meanwhile, whisk lemon zest, lemon juice, dill and black pepper essential oils and 2 Tbsp. oil in a large bowl; set vinaigrette aside.

Heat 3 Tbsp. oil in a large skillet over medium-high heat. Add beets, season with kosher salt and cook until browned, about 4 minutes per side. Transfer to bowl with vinaigrette, and toss to coat. Serve beets and dollops of yogurt drizzled with more oil, topped with more herbs, and seasoned with sea salt.

Heirloom Tomato Salad with Basil Oil

This simple salad requires the best quality tomatoes. Heirlooms are so beautiful! Choose different colors for a more colorful plate.

2 large heirloom tomatoes, sliced

1/4 cup extra virgin olive oil

2 drops basil essential oil

salt

pepper

fresh parsley for garnish (optional)

In a small measuring cup with a spout, combine the olive oil and essential oil. Arrange tomato slices on a large plate. Drizzle the olive oil mixture over the tomatoes, Sprinkle with desired amount of salt and pepper, to taste. Garnish with chopped fresh parsley (optional).

Egg Salad

10 hard-boiled eggs, diced

1 red, yellow, orange, or green bell pepper, diced very small

1 stalk celery, diced very small

½ cup mayonnaise

½ teaspoon salt

4 drops celery seed essential oil

4 drops black pepper essential oil

Combine the eggs, pepper, and celery in a medium bowl. In a small bowl, combine mayonnaise, salt, and oils. Gently combine the mayonnaise mixture with the egg mixture. Serve on a bed of greens, between bread slices, or as an open-faced sandwich.

EO Italian Vinaigrette

3 Tablespoons olive oil

2 Tablespoons white wine Vinegar

dash of salt

dash of black pepper

1 toothpick dip of oregano essential oil

1 toothpick dip of thyme essential oil

1 toothpick dip of marjoram essential oil

1 toothpick dip of basil essential oil

Combine first 4 ingredients, blending with a whisk. Add essential oils, using the toothpicks to stir the dressing. Makes 1/4 cup

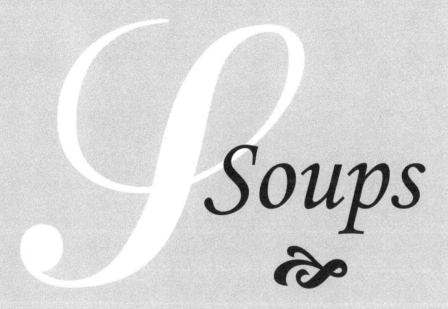

Soups

Tangy Cucumber Soup

2 pounds Persian or English cucumbers, halved lengthwise, seeded and chopped

1/2 cup plain fat-free Greek yogurt

3 tablespoons fresh lemon juice

2 small garlic cloves

1/2 cup extra-virgin olive oil, plus more for garnish

1 toothpick dip with dill essential oil, plus sprigs of fresh dill for garnish (optional)

kosher salt

2 drops black pepper essential oil

In a blender, puree the cucumbers, yogurt, lemon juice and garlic. With the machine on, gradually add the 1/2 cup of oil until incorporated. Add dill oil and season with salt and pepper. Cover and refrigerate until chilled, 30 minutes. Ladle the soup into bowls and garnish with a drizzle of olive oil and dill sprigs. This soup can also be served as a sauce for grilled meats or used as a salad dressing.

Spicy Pork and Beet Green Soup

This is hands down my favorite of all the soups I've ever made. It is so easy to make substitutions for several of the ingredients, making it very versatile. I guarantee you will keep coming back to this one!

½ pound ground pork sausage, of desired degree of spice (medium recommended)

1 clove garlic, finely chopped

4 cups low-sodium chicken broth

8 oz sliced oyster, shitake, or button mushrooms

1 bunch beet greens, (about 4 cups) You can also substitute mustard, kale, or turnip greens for the beet greens.

4 scallions, thinly sliced

2 tablespoons reduced-sodium soy sauce

1 teaspoon fish sauce (such as nam pla or nuoc nam)

8 oz. wide rice noodles (you can also use linguini, spaghetti, ramen noodles, etc)

2 drops ginger essential oil

3 drops black pepper essential oil

salt

Cook the sausage with the garlic in a large pot over medium-low heat, stirring and breaking up with a spoon, until browned and cooked through, 8–10 minutes. Drain the excess fat, though it is not necessary to remove it all. Add broth and bring to a boil; reduce heat and simmer 8–10 minutes. Add the mushrooms, beet greens, scallions, soy sauce, fish sauce, and pasta. Cook, stirring occasionally, until greens are tender and pasta is cooked through, about 8 minutes. Turn off the heat and add the ginger and black pepper oils. Season to taste with salt.

Moroccan Chicken and Butternut Squash Soup

1 tablespoon olive oil

1 cup chopped onion

3 (4-ounce) skinless, boneless chicken thighs, cut into bite-sized pieces

1 teaspoon ground cumin

1/8 to 1/4 teaspoon ground red pepper

3 cups (1/2-inch) cubed peeled butternut squash

2 tablespoons no-salt-added tomato paste

5 cups chicken stock

1/3 cup uncooked couscous

3/4 teaspoon kosher salt

1 zucchini, quartered lengthwise and sliced into 3/4-inch pieces

1 drop basil essential oil

2 drops orange essential oil

1 drop cinnamon essential oil

2 drops black pepper essential oil

Heat a Dutch oven over medium heat. Add olive oil to pan and swirl to coat. Add onion and cook for 4 minutes, stirring occasionally. Add chicken and cook for 4 minutes, browning on all sides. Add cumin and red pepper to pan; cook 1 minute, stirring constantly. Add butternut squash and tomato paste; cook 1 minute. Stir in chicken stock, scraping pan to loosen browned bits. Bring to a boil. Reduce heat and simmer 8 minutes. Stir in couscous, salt, and zucchini; cook 5 minutes or until squash is tender. Remove pan from heat. Stir in basil, orange, cinnamon and black pepper oils.

Spinach and Lentil Soup with Basil and Cheese

This recipe can be made ahead—just wait to stir in spinach and oils until after you reheat the soup.

1 tablespoon extra-virgin olive oil

1/4 cup chopped pancetta or bacon (about 1 ounce)

1 1/4 cups chopped onion

3/4 cup chopped celery

3/4 cup chopped carrot

1 bay leaf

1 cup dried brown lentils

3 cups fat-free, lower-sodium chicken broth

3 cups water

1 (6-ounce) package fresh baby spinach

1/4 cup (1 ounce) grated fresh parmesan cheese

2 drops lemon essential oil

1 drop thyme essential oil

1 drop basil essential oil

2 drops black pepper essential oil

Heat a Dutch oven over medium heat. Add olive oil to pan; swirl to coat. Add pancetta; cook 1 minute or until pancetta or bacon begins to brown, stirring occasionally. Add onion and next 3 ingredients (through bay leaf); cook 8 minutes or until vegetables are tender, stirring occasionally. Add lentils, broth, and 2 cups water; bring to a boil. Cover, reduce heat, and simmer 40 minutes or until lentils are tender and mixture is slightly thickened. Remove from heat. Discard bay leaf.

Place 2 cups lentil mixture in a blender. Remove the center piece of blender lid (to allow steam to escape), and secure blender lid on blender. Place a clean towel over opening in blender lid (to avoid splatters), and blend until smooth. Return pureed lentil mixture to pan. Add baby spinach, basil oil, parmesan cheese, lemon oil, thyme oil and black pepper oil; stir until spinach wilts. Serve immediately.

Mulligatawny Soup

6 tablespoons butter

1 cup onions diced

1 cup celery diced

1 apple, peeled, diced

1 tablespoon curry powder

3/4 cup flour (3 oz)

1 can coconut milk

6 cups chicken stock

2 tablespoons honey

2 teaspoons Sambal or sweet chili paste

2 cups of cooked rice, (about 1 cup uncooked)

3/4 lb. diced cooked chicken

2 drops ginger essential oil

4 drops lime essential oil

3 drops black pepper essential oil

salt to taste

In a 4qt stockpot melt butter. Add onions, celery, apples and salt. Cook over medium heat for 5 min. Add curry powder. Add flour stirring to coat the vegatables. Add chicken stock 1 cup at a time while whisking. Add the Sambal and honey. Simmer for 30min. Puree the soup. Add the cooked rice and chicken. Lastly, Add the ginger, lime, pepper oils. Salt to taste.

Sweet Potato Cauliflower Soup

1 large head cauliflower

olive oil for drizzling

few dashes garam masala (optional)

3 medium to large sized peeled sweet potatoes, cut into 1" pieces

1 sweet onion, diced

2 cloves garlic

3/4 teaspoons salt

7 cups water

3 drops black pepper essential oil

1 drop cinnamon essential oil

1 drop clove essential oil

1 drop ginger essential oil

salt

First, preheat your oven to 400 °F and cut up your cauliflower into bite sized pieces. Sprinkle cauliflower lightly with garam masala. Place cauliflower onto ungreased cookie sheet and lightly drizzle with olive oil. Place in oven and let roast until golden brown on the tops and tender, but not mushy (about 20-30 minutes.) There's no need to flip them. Just remove from oven and let cool while you cook the rest of the soup. In large stockpot, bring sweet potato, onion, garlic and water to a boil. Stir in salt. Reduce heat and allow to remain at a constant simmer until sweet potatoes are tender. Transfer soup to blender and puree until very smooth. Add the essential oils, then salt to taste. Warm up over stovetop if needed. Top with cooked cauliflower.

Minestrone with Chicken Meatballs

6 ounces ground chicken (about 3/4 cup)

1/2 cup fresh breadcrumbs

6 tablespoons finely grated Parmesan cheese, divided

4 garlic cloves minced

2 tablespoons chopped fresh chives

1 large egg, whisked to blend

2 tablespoons extra-virgin olive oil

1 leek, white and pale-green parts, sliced
   into 1/4-inch rounds

5 cups low-salt chicken broth

3/4 cup ditalini or other small pasta

1 cup sliced into 1/2-inch rounds peeled carrots

1 cup (packed) baby spinach

1 drop basil essential oil

1 drop thyme essential oil

2 drops black pepper essential oil

salt

Mix chicken, breadcrumbs, 3 tablespoons. parmesan, 2 minced garlic cloves, chives, egg, 3/4 tsp. salt, and 1/4 tsp. pepper in a medium bowl. Form into 1/2-inch-diameter meatballs (makes about 28). Heat oil in a small pot over medium heat. Cook meatballs until golden all over, about 3 minutes (they will finish cooking in soup). Transfer to a plate; set aside. Add leek to pot and cook, stirring often, until beginning to soften, about 3 minutes. Add 2 thinly sliced garlic cloves; cook for 1 minute. Add broth and 2 cups water; bring to a boil. Stir in pasta and carrots; simmer until pasta is almost al dente, about 8 minutes. Add meatballs; simmer until pasta is al dente, carrots are tender, and meatballs are cooked through, about 3 minutes. Add spinach and remaining 3 Tbsp. Parmesan; stir until spinach is wilted and Parmesan is melted. Season with basil, thyme , and black pepper oils. Season to taste with salt. Ladle soup into bowls. Garnish with parmesan cheese.

Potato, Cabbage, Leek Soup with Lemon Cream

1/2 cup sour cream

1 tablespoon fresh lemon juice

1/4 teaspoon finely grated lemon peel

2 tablespoons (1/4 stick) butter, divided

1 tablespoon extra-virgin olive oil

6 cups diced green cabbage (1/2-inch dice; from about 1/2 medium head)

3 cups chopped leeks (white and pale green parts only; 3 to 4 large)

3 large garlic cloves, pressed

3 cups 1/2-inch cubes peeled Yukon Gold potatoes (about 1 1/4 pounds)

1 2x2-inch piece Parmesan cheese rind (optional)

1 bay leaf

6 cups (or more) low-salt chicken broth

1 large carrot chopped

2 drops black pepper essential oil

2 drops carrot seed essential oil

2 drops celery seed essential oil

2 tablespoons chopped fresh chives (for garnish)

Whisk sour cream, lemon juice, and lemon peel in small bowl to blend. Cover and chill. Melt 1 tablespoon butter with 1 tablespoon olive oil in heavy large pot over medium-high heat. Add cabbage; sprinkle lightly with salt and freshly ground black pepper and sauté until cabbage is almost tender but not brown, 6 to 8 minutes. Using slotted spoon, transfer 1 cup cabbage to small bowl and reserve for garnish.

Add 1 tablespoon butter to pot with cabbage; add leeks, carrots and garlic. Sauté over medium heat until leeks soften slightly, about 3 minutes. Stir in potatoes, parmesan rind, (if desired) and bay leaf. Add 6 cups broth; bring to boil. Reduce heat to medium-low; cover and simmer until all vegetables are tender, 20 to 25 minutes. Discard Parmesan rind, if using, and bay leaf. Working in batches, puree soup in blender until smooth. Return puree to pot. Simmer until heated through, adding more broth by 1/4 cupfulls to thin soup to desired consistency. Season with salt and pepper oil, celery seed oil, carrot oil.

Ladle soup into bowls. Top each serving with some of reserved sautéed cabbage. Drizzle sour cream mixture over soup; sprinkle with chives and serve.

Butternut Squash Soup

2 tablespoons olive oil

2 onions, chopped

2 cloves of garlic, chopped

2 lbs butternut squash, peeled & cubed

4 cups vegetable broth

1 drop clove essential oil

3 drops nutmeg essential oil

1 drop cinnamon bark essential oil

salt

pepper

In soup pan, sauté onions, garlic, salt and pepper in olive oil over medium heat until tender. Add cubed squash and cook for 3-5 minutes. Next, add broth and bring to a boil. Boil on medium-high heat for 25 minutes or until squash is fork tender. Remove from heat. Using a hand mixer, puree until smooth. Stir in oils. Allow oils to infuse into soup for 5-8 minutes and then serve. Soup can be garnished with a spoonful of yogurt or sour cream.

Broccoli-Leek Soup with Parmesan

2 medium leeks, white and tender green parts only, finely chopped

1 1/2 pounds broccoli, stems peeled and sliced 1/2 inch thick, florets cut into 1-inch pieces

3 garlic cloves

5 cups chicken stock or canned low-sodium broth

salt to taste

1/2 cup sour cream

8 drops lemon essential oil

2 drops black pepper essential oil

1/4 cup snipped chives

1/4 cup grated Parmesan cheese

Steam the leeks, broccoli, and garlic until tender. Meanwhile, bring chicken stock to a boil in a stockpot. Add steamed vegetables to chicken stock. Remove from heat. Add sour cream, lemon and black pepper oils, and cheese.

Transfer the soup to a blender. Puree in batches until smooth. Ladle the soup into shallow bowls, Top with chives and serve.

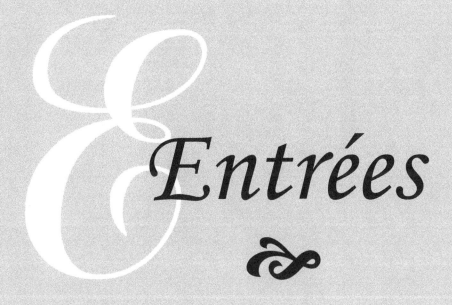

Entrées

Beef With Lemongrass & Rice Noodles

3 pounds boneless beef chuck, cut into 2" pieces

salt and freshly ground black pepper

4 cloves garlic chopped

2 teaspoons red pepper flakes

2 tablespoons vegetable oil

2 whole star anise pods

½ cup reduced-sodium soy sauce

1 tablespoon fish sauce
   (such as nam pla or nuoc nam)

¼ cup coconut or palm sugar

1 cup unsweetened coconut flakes

1 large onion, minced

1 pound carrots, peeled, cut into 2"
   lengths, halved if large

4 scallions, cut into 1" lengths,
   plus more for serving (thinly sliced)

8 oz. rice vermicelli noodles

4 drops lemongrass essential oil

2 drops ginger essential oil

lime wedges (for serving)

Season beef with salt and pepper. Heat oil in a large Dutch oven over medium-high heat. Working in batches, cook beef, turning occasionally, until browned, 10–15 minutes; transfer to a plate. Combine the star anise, soy sauce, fish sauce, palm sugar, beef along with any juices, and 10 cups water in the dutch oven. Bring to a boil, reduce heat, and simmer, partially covered, until beef is tender and liquid is slightly thickened, 2½–3 hours.

Meanwhile, preheat oven to 350°F. Toast coconut flakes on a rimmed baking sheet, tossing occasionally, until golden around the edges, about 4 minutes; set aside. Use a slotted spoon to find and remove the star anise pods. Add onions and carrots to stew and cook, partially covered, until vegetables are soft and beef is falling apart, 35–45 minutes. Mix in scallions (they should wilt slightly). Meanwhile, cook noodles according to package directions. Combine rice noodles with beef. Stir in lemongrass and ginger essential oils. Top with toasted coconut and sliced scallions. Serve with lime wedges.

Pan Fried Cod With Spicy Tomato Sauce

6 garlic cloves, coarsely chopped

2 teaspoons smoked paprika

1 1/2 teaspoons ground cumin

1/2 teaspoon cayenne pepper

2 tablespoons tomato paste

2 tablespoons fresh lemon juice

2 teaspoons sugar

1/2 teaspoon salt

8 tablespoons (or more) sunflower oil, divided

4 6oz. cod fillets (preferably wild) or other mild fish

salt and freshly ground black pepper

2 toothpick dips cinnamon essential oil

2 drops black pepper essential oil

2 tablespoons chopped fresh cilantro

lemon wedges

Purée garlic, smoked paprika, cumin, cayenne, cinnamon, and 6 Tbsp. oil in a small food processor, adding more oil by teaspoonfuls to garlic paste if needed. Add garlic paste to large skillet. Cook, stirring constantly for 30 seconds. Carefully (mixture will splatter) add tomato paste and 1/2 cup water to the garlic paste. Bring to a simmer; continue simmering for 30 seconds. Stir in lemon juice, sugar and salt. Remove from heat. Be sure the sauce is no longer simmering and stir in the essential oils. Heat 2 tablespoons oil in a large heavy skillet over medium-high heat. Season the fish with salt and pepper. Working in 2 batches, cook fish until golden, 1-2 minutes per side. Arrange fish over tomato sauce. Sprinkle cilantro over. Serve with lemon wedges alongside.

Spinach and Mozzarella Stuffed Chicken

4 boneless, skinless chicken breasts

2 cloves garlic, cracked

2 cups whole milk

1 drop black pepper essential oil

1 drop thyme essential oil

1 cup fresh baby spinach

1 cup shredded mozzarella cheese

2 tablespoons butter

2 tablespoons olive oil

1 Ib wheat spaghetti

Toothpicks

Place chicken breasts in the center of a plastic food storage bag. Pound out the chicken from the center of the bag outward using a mallet, until about 1/4 inch thick. Add garlic and thyme and pepper essential oils to the milk in a medium bowl. Add chicken, and cover with plastic wrap. Refrigerate for 1 hour.

Meanwhile preheat oven to 375 °F. Pat chicken dry, then season with salt. Divide spinach and mozzarella between chicken breasts. Starting at the longest end of the chicken, roll the flattened chicken breast tightly, forming a roulade. Use toothpicks to hold it together. Place butter and olive oil in a nonstick skillet over moderate heat. When skillet is hot, sear stuffed chicken until golden on all sides. Finish in oven for 10 minutes.

Meanwhile, cook pasta according to directions on the package.

To make the sauce:
add all ingredients to blender until smooth. Add sauce to cooked pasta. After removing the chicken from the oven, remove the toothpicks. Top the pasta with chicken. Garnish with parmesan and parsley.

SAUCE:

2 pints cherry tomatoes

2 tablespoons tomato paste

2 cloves garlic

1 shallot

1 drop thyme essential oil

1 drop black pepper essential oil

1 drop basil essential oil

1/8 cup chopped, fresh parsley

1/2 cup grated Parmesan cheese

Conchiglie with Chickpeas, Garlic, and Rosemary

1 medium onion, quartered

1 medium carrot, peeled,
   cut into 1-inch pieces

1 celery stalk, cut into 1-inch pieces

6 garlic cloves, (4 whole, 2 chopped)

1/2 cup flat-leaf parsley leaves

1/2 teaspoon crushed red pepper flakes

1/2 cup olive oil, divided

salt

2 tablespoons tomato paste

2 15-ounce cans chickpeas, rinsed

1 pound Conchigile (small shells)
   or elbow macaroni

1 tablespoon fresh rosemary

2 drops rosemary essential oil

2 drops black pepper essential oil

1 drop basil essential oil

Pulse onion, carrot, celery, whole garlic cloves, parsley, and red pepper flakes in a food processor until finely chopped; transfer to a small bowl and set aside. Wipe out food processor bowl and set aside. Heat 1/4 cup oil in a large heavy pot over medium heat; add reserved vegetable mixture, season with salt, and cook, stirring often, until golden, 8-10 minutes. Stir tomato paste and 1 cup water in a small bowl to combine; add to pot. Cook, scraping up any browned bits from bottom of pot. Bring to a boil, reduce heat, and simmer until liquid has almost evaporated, 5-8 minutes. Add chickpeas and 2 cups water to pot and simmer for 15 minutes to let flavors meld. Transfer 1 cup chickpea mixture to food processor; purée until smooth, then stir back into sauce to thicken. Meanwhile, cook pasta in a large pot of boiling salted water, stirring occasionally, until al dente. Drain pasta, reserving 1 1/2 cups pasta cooking liquid. Add rosemary, pepper and basil oils. Add pasta and 1/2 cup pasta cooking liquid to sauce and stir to coat. Increase heat to medium and continue stirring, adding more pasta cooking liquid as needed, until sauce coats pasta. Heat remaining 1/4 cup oil in a small saucepan over medium-low heat; add chopped garlic and rosemary and cook until sizzling stops, about 1 minute. Divide pasta among bowls and drizzle with garlic-rosemary oil.

Bacon and Leek Risotto with Poached Egg

5 cups low-salt chicken broth

2 drops thyme essential oil

2 drops black pepper essential oil

1 tablespoon olive oil

6 slices thick-cut bacon, cut crosswise into 1/2-inch pieces

2 cups thinly sliced leeks
   (white and pale green parts only; about 2 large)

1 1/2 cups arborio rice or medium-grain white rice
   (about 10 ounces)

3/4 cup dry white wine

3 tablespoons finely chopped fresh Italian parsley

1 tablespoon butter

2 tablespoons finely grated Parmesan cheese

fresh Italian parsley leaves (for garnish)

additional finely grated Parmesan cheese (for garnish)

6 large eggs

salt

Bring chicken broth to a simmer in medium saucepan. Add the thyme and black pepper oils. Remove from heat. Cover to keep warm. Heat oil in heavy large saucepan over medium heat. Add bacon and cook until crisp, stirring occasionally. Using slotted spoon, transfer bacon to paper towels to drain. Add leeks to drippings in pan; cook until soft but not brown, stirring often, 4 to 5 minutes. Transfer 2 generous tablespoonfuls leeks to small bowl; reserve for garnish. Add rice to pan; stir 1 to 2 minutes. Add wine; stir until absorbed, about 2 minutes. Add 1 cup warm broth to saucepan; stir until broth is absorbed. Repeat adding broth and stirring until rice is tender but still firm to bite and sauce is creamy, stirring almost constantly, about 23 minutes total. Add bacon, chopped parsley, butter, and 2 tablespoons cheese. Season to taste with salt. Bring large skillet of water just to simmer over medium-low heat. Sprinkle water with salt. Working with 1 egg at a time, crack into small bowl and slide egg into simmering water. Cook eggs until whites are cooked through but yolks are still runny, 3 to 4 minutes. Remove each egg using slotted spoon, and set aside. Divide risotto among 6 bowls. Top risotto in each bowl with 1 poached egg. Sprinkle egg with salt . Sprinkle with parsley leaves, additional cheese, and reserved leeks over each serving.

Roasted Cauliflower with Lentils and Spinach

1 cup green lentils, rinsed

2 cup water

1 head of cauliflower, cut into 1- to 1 1/2-inch florets

1/4 cup plus 1 tablespoon extra-virgin olive oil

1/4 teaspoon ground cumin

pinch of cayenne

salt & freshly ground pepper

2 tablespoons tahini

3 tablespoons fresh lemon juice

1 teaspoon honey

1 drop cinnamon essential oil

1 drop ginger essential oil

10 dates, pitted and chopped

1/2 small red onion, sliced thin

3 cups loosely packed spinach or arugula

Preheat the oven to 425°F. On a large rimmed baking sheet, toss the cauliflower with the 1/4 cup of olive oil, the cumin, and cayenne. Season with salt and pepper.

Roast for 20 minutes, turning, until the cauliflower is tender and golden brown. Meanwhile in a saucepan, combine the lentils with 2 cups of water and bring to a boil. Simmer over moderate heat until tender, 20 minutes.

Drain well and let cool. In a large bowl, whisk the tahini with the lemon juice, honey, essential oils, the remaining 1 tablespoon of olive oil and 2 tablespoons of water until smooth. Add the lentils and season with salt and pepper; toss to coat. Scrape the roasted cauliflower into the bowl and add the dates, onion and spinach. Toss the salad, transfer to a platter or bowls and serve.

Stuffed Tomatoes with Chicken

6 vine-ripened tomatoes

1/2 lb. ground chicken

1 cup bread crumbs

2 clove garlic, minced

4 drops thyme essential oil

2 drops black pepper essential oil

1 cup grated Parmesan cheese

1/4 cup olive oil

salt

Preheat oven to 400 °F. Slice tomatoes in half horizontally and scoop out pulp and seeds. Salt insides, Meanwhile, in a medium bowl, mix together bread crumbs, chicken, garlic, pepper oil, basil oil , 1/2 cup of the grated Parmesan and salt . Stuff tomatoes with the filling, sprinkle with remaining Parmesan, and bake until tomatoes are cooked through and tops are golden brown, about 30 minutes.

Shrimp Skewers with Fresh Mango Chutney

FOR SHRIMP:

1/4 cup vegetable oil

2 tablespoons fresh lime juice

1(1-inch) piece fresh jalapeño, chopped (about 2 tsp)

1(1-inch) piece peeled ginger, chopped

1 large garlic clove, smashed

2 teaspoons ground garam masala (Indian spice blend)

3/4 teaspoon turmeric

1 drop nutmeg essential oil

1 drop ginger essential oil

2 lb large uncooked, peeled shrimp

FOR CHUTNEY:

1 teaspoon ground cumin

1(3/4-lb) mango, chopped

1/3 seedless cucumber, peeled and chopped (3/4 cup)

1/2 cup chopped red onion

1 to 2 teaspoons minced fresh jalapeño with seeds

3 tablespoons fresh lime juice

3 tablespoons thinly sliced mint

3 tablespoons chopped cilantro

MARINATE SHRIMP:
Purée all ingredients for marinating shrimp, except shrimp, with 1/2 teaspoon salt in a blender until smooth. Pour into a sealable bag, then add shrimp and marinate at cool room temperature, turning bag occasionally, 30 minutes.

MAKE CHUTNEY WHILE SHRIMP MARINATES:
Toast cumin in a dry small skillet over medium heat, stirring occasionally, until fragrant, about 1 minute. Stir together remaining chutney ingredients with 1/4 tsp salt, in a small bowl. Then sprinkle with toasted cumin.

FOR THE KEBABS:
Cook in a hot well-oiled large (2-burner) ridged grill pan under a broiler, turning once, about 5 minutes total. Thread 4 shrimp onto each skewer, leaving small spaces between them. Put on a tray. Serve with chutney.

Homemade Alfredo Sauce

1 pint heavy cream

1/2 cup (1 stick) unsalted butter, softened

1 cup freshly grated Parmesan

1 drop black pepper essential oil

1 drop nutmeg essential oil

Chopped fresh flat-leaf parsley, for garnish. Heat heavy cream over low-medium heat. Add butter and whisk to melt. Remove from heat. Sprinkle in cheese and stir. Add black pepper and nutmeg oils. Add salt to taste. Serve with pasta. Serve immediately. Garnish with chopped parsley.

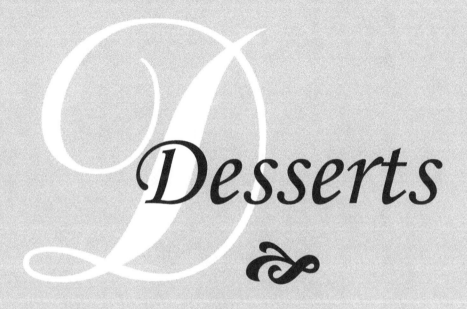

Desserts

Raw Brownies No Bake

1 1/2 cups walnuts

pinch sea salt

1/2 cup dates, pitted

1/3 cup unsweetened cocoa powder

1 teaspoon vanilla extract

2 drops cinnamon essential oil

Place walnuts and salt in a food processor. Process until finely ground. Add remaining ingredients and process until all mixed and uniformly crumbly. With the machine running, add a few drops of water at a time, just until the mass starts to stick together in a big ball. Roll mixture into balls or press into a square pan and cut into squares. Balls or squares can then be rolled in dried coconut, chopped nuts, or cocoa powder if you wish.

Flour Free Oatmeal Cookies

These cookies remind us of a chewy granola bar. It is versatile in the way that you can add other things in to the batter. We made them with pecans and chocolate chips, for example. You could also add seeds, dried wolfberries, and other nuts. Just add them in small amounts or the batter won't hold together.

1/3 cup unsalted butter

7/8 cup (6 oz brown sugar)

1/2 teaspoon salt

2 drops cinnamon essential oil

1 drop nutmeg essential oil

1 drop clove essential oil

1/2 teaspoon baking powder

1 1/2 teaspoons vanilla extract

2 teaspoons raw apple cider vinegar (or white)

2 large eggs

2 1/2 cups (8 3/4 ounces) rolled oats

In a large bowl, beat together the butter, sugar, salt, oils, baking powder, vanilla, and vinegar until light and fluffy. Add the eggs one at a time. Beating well after each egg is added. Stir in the oats. Cover bowl and refrigerate for about 1 hour. Preheat the oven to 375 °F. Lightly grease or line with parchment, 2 baking sheets. Remove the dough from the refrigerator, and drop it by the tablespoon full onto the prepared baking sheets. Flatten each cookie to about ¼" thick using your fingers that have been moistened with water. Bake the cookies for 10 minutes, or until their edges are lightly browned. They will not look completely done in the center but that is fine. Remove them from the oven and allow the cookies to cool on the baking sheet for about 5 minutes before transferring them to a cooling rack to cool completely.

Yuzu Wafer Candy

You can substitute any of your favorite flavors of essential oils! Also, this makes a fairly large batch, so feel free to cut it in half if not making it for a large group.

2 cups raw organic sugar
7 tablespoons water, divided
3/4 teaspoon cream of tartar
6 drops yuzu essential oil

Remove 3 tablespoons of the sugar and put in a small bowl. Put the rest of the sugar and 6 tablespoons of the water in a large saucepan and bring to a boil. Set a timer and boil for 3 minutes, then remove from the fire. Combine the cream of tartar, the last tablespoon of water and the yuzu oil with the 3 tablespoons of sugar in the bowl. Add this to the boiled mixture and stir gently for 3 minutes, or until it begins to take shape. It sets up very quickly at this point.

Drop by the teaspoonful into plastic candy molds or onto waxed paper. Let cool completely before serving. Lasts about 2 weeks in an airtight container.

Watermelon Granita

4 cups (1 3/4lb.) cubed seedless watermelon

¼ cup agave nectar

10 drops lime essential oil

Puree all ingredients in a blender until smooth. Pour into a 9x9x2" metal baking pan. Freeze mixture for one hour. Stir, mashing any frozen parts with the back of a fork. Cover and freeze mixture until firm, about 2 hours. Using a fork, scrape granita to form icy flakes. Granita can be stored for around 5 days covered tightly with foil and kept frozen. Flake with a fork some more before serving. Enjoy!

Orange Cardamom Cookies

COOKIE DOUGH:

1 3/4 cups (7 1/2 ounces) All-Purpose flour

1/2 teaspoon baking powder

1/4 teaspoon baking soda

1 1/2 teaspoons ground cardamom or 2 drops
   YL cardamom essential oil

1/4 teaspoon salt

3/4 cup (1 1/2 sticks, 6 ounces) unsalted butter,
   room temperature

1 cup (7 ounces) sugar

zest from 2 small oranges

2 tablespoons (1 ounces) orange juice

2 large eggs

GLAZE:

1 cup (4 ounces) powdered sugar

2 tablespoons (1 ounce) water

10 drops orange essential oil

Preheat your oven to 350 °F. Grease baking sheets or line with parchment. Whisk together flour, baking powder, baking soda, cardamom, & salt; set aside in a large bowl or stand mixer, mix together the butter, sugar, and orange zest until smooth. Add the orange juice and eggs. Beat until combined. Gradually add the flour mixture and beat until combined. Scoop 1 1/4" balls of dough onto the prepared baking sheets, leaving 2 inches between each cookie (these spread quite a bit). Flatten slightly with the palm of your hand. Bake for 14-16 minutes, or until the cookies are set and are starting to brown. Remove them from the oven and cool on the sheet pan until they're set enough to move without breaking. Repeat with remaining dough. While they are cooling, whisk the powdered sugar, water, and orange essential oil until fully combined and smooth. Brush or drizzle the glaze onto the cookies and allow to harden fully until storing them in an airtight container for up to 5 days. Makes about 2 dozen cookies.

Coconut Macaroons with Rose

For all you lovers of rose out there!

2 1/2 cups unsweetened shredded coconut

4 large egg whites

2/3 cup sugar

1 teaspoon vanilla extract

1-2 drops rose essential oil (depending on desired strength. One drop is very subtle.)

fine sugar for coating

Cook first 3 ingredients in a medium sauce- pan over low heat, stirring occasionally, until mixture is hot, dry to the touch, and starts pulling away from sides of pan, about 15 minutes.

Scrape dough into a heatproof bowl. Stir in vanilla and rose essential oil. Press plastic wrap on top of dough. Chill for at least 5 hours or overnight.

Preheat oven to 300°F. Line a baking sheet with parchment paper or a silicone baking mat. If you'd like, you can stack it on top of a second sheet (this keeps cookie bottoms from browning too quickly).

Roll 1 tablespoon of dough into a ball. Dip into white sanding sugar. Repeat with remaining dough. Bake cookies until lightly golden on top and slightly firm to the touch, 25-30 minutes. Let the cookie sheet cool on a wire rack.

Gingerbread Cupcakes with Cinnamon Cream Cheese

1 3/4 cups (7 1/4ounces) Whole Wheat Flour

1 teaspoon baking soda

2 drops cinnamon bark essential oil

2 drops ginger essential oil

2 drops clove essential oil

2 drops nutmeg essential oil

1/4 teaspoon salt

1/2 cup (8 tablespoons, 4 ounces) unsalted butter, melted

1/2 cup (3 3/4 ounces) organic brown sugar

1/2 cup (6 ounces) molasses

1 large egg

1/2 cup water

FROSTING:

6 tablespoons unsalted butter, at room temperature

8-ounce package cream cheese, softened

4 cups (16 ounces) organic confectioners' sugar

2 drops cinnamon bark essential oil

1 to 2 tablespoons organic milk,

   enough to make a spreadable frosting

Note: If you would like to see cinnamon specks it the frosting, add a dash of ground cinnamon. Preheat the oven to 350°F. Lightly grease a 12-cup muffin tin or line with cupcake papers. To make the cupcakes: Combine the flour, baking soda, and salt. Set aside.

Whisk together the melted butter, brown sugar, molasses, and egg, add the cinnamon, ginger, clove, & nutmeg essential oils. Add 1/4 cup of the water, then half the dry mixture, and stir. Add the remaining water and dry mixture, stirring until thoroughly combined. Spoon the batter into the prepared pan. Bake the cupcakes for 22 to 25 minutes, until a toothpick inserted in the center of one comes out clean. Remove the cupcakes from the oven, and transfer them to a rack to cool for 30 minutes. To make the frosting: Beat together the butter and cream cheese until light and fluffy. Add the sugar and cinnamon oil, beating well. Add the milk a little at a time, until the frosting is spreadable. Fill a piping bag with the frosting, and pipe large swirls on top of the cooled cupcakes or simply frost by hand. Makes 12 cupcakes.

Homemade Frankincense Marshmallows

We love the taste of frankincense. These turned out fabulous, and people who don't know frankincense loved the flavor! It's a fun project, and you will feel very proud when others sample your marshmallows! There is no reason why you can't swap out the frankincense for any of your other favorite essential oils.

3 packages (1/4-ounce each) unflavored gelatin

1 cup (8 ounces) cool water, divided

1 1/2 cups (10 1/2 ounces) granulated organic raw sugar

1 cup (11 ounces) Non-GMO light corn syrup

1/8 teaspoon salt

1 teaspoon vanilla extract

3 drops frankincense (we used Sacred Frankincense)

confectioners' sugar, to sprinkle on top

Combine the gelatin and 1/2 cup cool water in the bowl of an electric mixer fitted with the whisk attachment. Combine the sugar, corn syrup, salt, and 1/2 cup cool water in a small, deep saucepan. Cook the mixture over medium heat, stirring, until the sugar dissolves. Raise the heat to high and cook, without stirring, until the syrup reaches 240°F on a candy thermometer (soft ball stage). Remove from the heat. With mixer on low speed, slowly pour the sugar syrup into the softened gelatin. Increase the speed to high, and whip until the mixture is very thick and fluffy, and has cooled to lukewarm, 8 to 10 minutes. (It should be cool enough that you can spread it into the pan without burning your fingers.) Add vanilla and frankincense towards the end of the mixing time. Spread the marshmallow mixture into a greased 9" x 13" pan (glass or ceramic is best). Use your wet hands to smooth and flatten the marshmallows. Sprinkle confectioners' sugar over the top, and let sit for several hours (or overnight) before cutting. Use a greased knife or cookie cutters to make squares or other shapes. Yield: about 100 1" squares. Toss finished shapes in sifted confectioner's sugar.

Fudgy Brownies with Cassia Essential Oil

We've had a lot of great feedback with these brownies!! The cassia is the secret ingredient that makes people say: "What is that flavor? It's awesome!".

3/4 cup (6 oz) unsalted butter

2 cups (14 oz) sugar

1 cup (3 oz) Dutch process cocoa powder

1 teaspoon salt

1/2 teaspoon baking powder

1 tablespoon vanilla extract

1 drop cassia essential oil

3 large eggs

1 cup (4 1/4 oz) unbleached all-purpose flour

1 cup (4 oz) chopped walnuts or pecans

1 cup (6 oz) chocolate chips (optional)

Preheat oven to 325 °F. Lightly grease a 9"x13" pan. In a medium saucepan, melt the butter over low heat, then add the sugar and stir to combine. Return the mixture to the heat, briefly, just until it's hot (110 degrees F - 120 degrees F), but not bubbling; it will become shiny looking as you stir it. Heating this mixture a second time will dissolve more of the sugar, which will make a shiny crust on top of the brownies. Remove pan from heat. Stir in the cocoa, salt, baking powder, vanilla & cassia. Wisk in the eggs, stirring until smooth, then add the flour and nuts and chips, again stirring until smooth. Spoon the batter into the prepared pan.

Bake brownies for 29 to 32 minutes, until a toothpick inserted in the center comes out clean, or with just a tiny amount of crumb clinging to it. The edges of the brownies should be set, but the center still soft. Remove the brownies from the oven and cool on a rack before cutting and serving. Makes 2 dozen 2-inch brownies.

Lavender Shortbread

6 3/8oz unsalted butter, at room temperature

1/2 cup organic cane sugar

1 3/4 cups + 3 tablespoons all-purpose flour.

1/2 teaspoon salt

1/2 teaspoon vanilla extract

3 drops lavender essential oil

extra sugar for dusting the tops (optional)

Beat butter in a stand mixer on medium-low speed until smooth. Add the sugar and salt and mix on medium-low speed for about 2 minutes, until fluffy looking. Scrape down the bottom and sides of the bowl with a rubber spatula. Add vanilla and lavender essential oil on low speed for about 30 seconds. Add the flour in 2 additions, mixing on low speed until just combined. Mound the dough on a piece of plastic wrap on a work surface. Wrap dough with the plastic wrap as loosely as possible. Use your hands to pack down the dough into a ¼ inch thick rectangle. Refrigerate for at least 2 hours, or up to 1 month.

Preheat oven to 325 °F. Remove the dough from the refrigerator. Line a large baking sheet with parchment paper (or 2 sheets if you roll the dough thin for thin, crisp cookies.). Unwrap the dough and use a rolling pin to roll out to desired thickness and to smooth out the tops. The dough may crack on the edges but that's okay. You can use your fingers to smooth it out. Cut shortbread into squares or rectangles, using all of the dough. If you are dusting with granulated sugar, do this now. If the dough has gotten too soft, put it back in the refrigerator until stiff again. Place cookies on the prepared baking sheet, leaving ¾" between them and bake for 17-19 minutes in a standard oven (a little less in convection) or until pale golden brown. Rotate sheet pan halfway through cooking time. Cool cookies on the baking sheet for 5-10 minutes, then transfer to a cooling rack to cool completely. Store in an airtight container for up to 3 days.

Nut Crusts

These are a wonderful base for many different fillings. Below is a recipe for an apple filling we made to go with them. But possibilities are nearly endless! How about fresh diced strawberries in agave with whipped cream on top?

2 cups of pecans, walnuts, or almonds (or combination)

3 tablespoons agave nectar

1 teaspoon ground ginger or 1 drop ginger essential oil

2 tablespoons whole wheat flour

1/2 teaspoon salt

2 teaspoons organic cold-pressed coconut oil plus more for greasing the pan

Grease 1 standard 12-cup muffin tin or 24-cup mini muffin tin with coconut oil. Add nuts to a food processor and process until coarsely ground. Add the remaining ingredients and process until a coarse dough forms. Gather into 1 large ball. Grab tablespoon sized pieces if you are using the standard muffin cups, and teaspoon sized pieces for the mini muffin cups. Press the dough firmly into the bottom and up the sides of each cup. Chill dough for 1 hour. Meanwhile, heat your oven to 350 °F. Bake until firm, about 8- 10 minutes. Let the pan cool on a wire rack for about 10 minutes before removing the crusts from the pan. Store in an airtight container. Use within 3 days.

Apple Filling for Nut Crusts

2 large Gala apples, diced very small

3 tablespoons honey

¼ teaspoon salt

1 toothpick dip of clove essential oil

1-2 drops cinnamon essential oil

1 drop nutmeg essential oil

ground cinnamon (optional)

flakey sea salt (optional)

Combine apples, salt and honey in a small saucepan or skillet, cook on medium-low heat until apples are soft, about 4 minutes. Remove from heat and add the essential oils. Spoon the filling into crusts. Sprinkle ground cinnamon and flakey sea salt over each tart as garnish if desired. These may be refrigerated up to 3 days.

Honey & Nutmeg Ice Cream or Lavender Ice Cream

You can change this to lavender ice cream by using 1/3 cup sugar instead of the honey, and adding 4 drops lavender essential oil instead of the nutmeg.

4 egg yolks

1 cup whole milk

1/8 teaspoon salt

7 tablespoons raw honey

1 ½ cups heavy cream

2 drops nutmeg essential oil

In a medium bowl, whisk egg yolks then set aside. In a medium saucepan over medium heat, whisk together the milk and salt. Heat until milk is steaming, just before it begins to boil. Remove from heat, then slowly drizzle the warm milk into the egg yolks, whisking constantly to temper the eggs. Return the milk and egg mixture to the saucepan and cook on low heat, whisking frequently until the custard mixture becomes the consistency of warm pudding. Remove from heat and strain through a fine mesh strainer into a medium bowl, to remove any lumps. While the mixture is still warm, whisk in the honey until dissolved. Whisk in the nutmeg essential oil and heavy cream. Cover the bowl with plastic wrap, and refrigerate for at least 4 hours, or overnight. Follow the directions on your ice cream machine to churn the custard until smooth and thick. Eat it immediately, or chill in the freezer before serving. Use within 5 days.

Dairy-Free Lavender Ice Cream

Feel free to substitute the lavender in this recipe for another oil of your choice. Be sure to use full-fat coconut milk, this will help make it creamier.

1 14 ounce can coconut milk

1 1/2 cups almond milk or other non-dairy milk

3 tablespoons organic sugar

4 drops lavender essential oil

Put all the ingredients in a blender and puree until smooth. Refrigerate mixture for a least an hour or so, until cold. Follow the directions on your ice cream machine to churn the mixture until thick. Eat right away or freeze until hardened.

Jason and Britney Pilkington, gastronomists, have many years of combined experience traveling in the search of delicious food and drink and now they have shared some of their best finds in creative cooking with the rest of us.

They have combined their love of pure essential oils, a desire to find more ways to use them in daily life and married that knowledge with the pursuit of creative food ideas and presentation, first through recipes on Jason's website and now the offering of this cookbook for creatively using essential oils in cooking.

Jason and Britney are raising their young family to place value on our environment and are being mindful of passing the lost understanding of the benefits of essential oils to the next generation by using the oils every day at home. Their fresh ideas and recipes can get you started in developing your own creativity, and of course their ultimate goal is to help you begin using pure essential oils in new ways every day.

Jason and Britney reside in Virginia along with their two children.

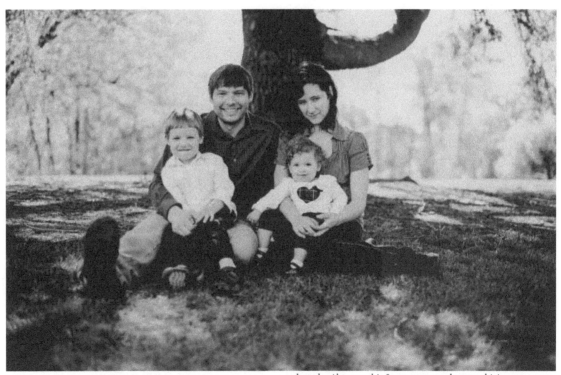

photo by Abercrombie Imagery www.abercrombieimagery.com

Mail Order Form

A Chef's Guide to Cooking with Essential Oils
(by – Jason & Britney Pilkington)

Single Copy and Bulk Pricing
You can order individual copies through our website:
www.ScentfanaticPublishing.com

____ Single copies .... $11.95 (per copy) _____

____ 5-Pack – Special ($10.95 each) .... $54.75 (per pack) _____

____ 10-Pack – Special ($9.95 each) .... $99.50 (per pack) _____

____ 15-Pack – Special ($8.95 each) .... $134.25 (per pack) _____

____ 20-Pack – Special ($7.95 each) .... $159.00 (per pack) _____

Subtotal _____

S&H (US: 10% - $3.99 min.) _____

Total _____

Name:_____

Address:_____

City:_____ State: _____ Zip: _____

Phone: (_____) _____ _____

Email: _____

Check or Money Orders Only
Payable to: Jason Pilkington

Mail to:
**Jason Pilkington
202 Charity Lane
Gladstone, VA 24553**